The Complete Guide to Losing Weight

Recipes Low-Carb

Author

Sharon K. Browning

The Low Carb Diet (Part 1) Introduction to the Low Carb Diet (Chapter 1)

The Diet in Context

Low-carbohydrate or low-carb diets are gaining popularity in today's dieting world. Low carb diets are defined in a number of ways; some propose that the limit is set at less than 20% of your total calorie intake, while others advocate a general decrease in carb consumption.

Regardless of the criteria, all low carb diets advise you to cut down on carbs, particularly if you want to lose weight.

The link between carbs, calories, and fats is the key to the low carb diet's success. Carbohydrates, like other dietary types, are turned into calories when ingested. These calories are supposed to be used as fuel for the body's normal processes.

You burn more calories if you live an active lifestyle. Calories you don't consume are stored as fat, which serves as a backup fuel source for later usage.

The feeding behaviors of a bear are one of the greatest instances of this connection. A bear will devour much more food than he needs prior to the winter season. This is because hunting will be tough for the bear throughout the winter. The bear will store the food he eats as fat in order to keep his body fed and functioning. Instead of eating, his body will utilise stored fat while he hibernates.

Today's issue is that the ordinary person's lifestyle is gradually becoming more sedentary. This indicates that if a person keeps their carb consumption the same but lowers their physical activity, more carbohydrates are converted into calories that aren't utilised. Fat is accumulated in proportion to the number of calories that are not utilised. This is where a low-carbohydrate diet may help to alleviate the issue. Carbohydrate consumption must be restricted to compensate for the reduction in calorie intake.

Doctors, dietitians, and other health experts are now recommending the low carb diet to patients with a variety of ailments. High blood pressure, diabetes, and cardiac difficulties are examples of these disorders.

Advantages and Drawbacks

Aside from the health advantages, such as illness prevention and management, people who follow the low carb diet's suggested meal patterns have been shown to boost their appearance. In fact, many are more interested in the weight reduction advantages than the real health benefits.

Weight loss is achievable because carbohydrate consumption is controlled, which reduces the creation of fat. You may even burn undesirable fat if you combine this diet with an active lifestyle. Weight loss becomes even more probable and quicker with the reduction of fat creation and the burning up of previously stored fat in your body.

Your muscles develop stronger as well as your body becomes slimmer. The logical companion to a low-carb diet is a high-protein diet. This implies that not only will you be able to lose weight, but you will also be able to tone and define your muscles. The ultimate effect is twofold: your body will not only look amazing, but it will also have increased strength and endurance. The stronger you are, the more active your lifestyle may be, and the more endurance you have, the longer your activities can be performed. This combination provides the ideal situation: a diet that not only makes your body look nice, but also makes it feel well and perform well.

Another advantage is that, contrary to its name, it does not completely prevent you from consuming carbohydrates. Rather, it just reduces your carb consumption. This means you can continue to eat your favorite carbs. This diet may nevertheless provide taste, flavor, and a sensation of fullness. Another reason why most individuals prefer the low-carb diet to others is because of this. Some diets completely exclude particular food categories, sacrificing flavor and enjoyment in the process. You don't have to get hungry on a low-carb diet. In fact, the food tastes better, in addition to being healthier options.

However, there are certain drawbacks to a low-carb diet. The first is the period of adjustment. During the first several weeks of the diet, you may find yourself easily exhausted. This is due to the fact that your calorie supply has shrunk. This is a transitory effect, and after your body has acclimated to the diet, you will feel more invigorated since your digestive system is now digesting the quantity of food it is supposed to digest. Your absorption improves, and your metabolism stabilizes.

Another issue is the higher cost of some of the diet's suggested items. The low carb diet, for example, suggests salmon instead of any other fish. You must use the slimmer or choice cut varieties of meat or poultry instead of any other portion of the animal. On the other hand, you may still choose for the less expensive but still low-carb options. For example, instead of salmon, you may choose tilapia, a white fish known as "the poor man's fish."

Take notice that, like any other diet, the low carb diet is not intended to replace any physical activity or medicine you may be taking. Diets are supposed to supplement, not replace, your existing health habits. Diets are most effective when used in combination with other healthy lifestyle choices. If you combine a low-carb diet with regular exercise, you may easily achieve your ideal weight. If you want to follow this diet, talk to your doctor beforehand, particularly if you have any medical issues.

Chapter 2: Weight Loss and Low-Carb Food Groups

Food Groups with Low Carbohydrates

Take this list to the store with you on your next shopping trip and make informed decisions. The following foods have some of the lowest carbohydrate levels. Make these components the foundation of your meals.

These are the foods:

For fruits and veggies Zucchini

Cauliflower\sMushrooms Squash, celery, cherry tomatoes

For fish and fruits

Avocado Strawberries Peaches Cantaloupe Watermelon Tilapia Catfish

Halibut For poultry, salmon Thighs of chicken

In the case of flesh

Chicken breasts with ground turkey

Steak sirloin Tenderloin of pork Beef roast For other food products,

Eggs

Plain Walnuts, Cottage Cheese, Greek Yogurt Almond Jerky

flour

Food Groups High in Protein

The following are some foods that are rich in protein: Cottage cheese is a kind of cheese that is made

Yogurt from Greece

Eggs Steak with Milk

Beef patty Breast of chicken Breast of turkey Tilapia

Halibut with tuna and salmon

Anchovies\sSardines Peanuts Almonds Chorizo Bacon

Seeds from a watermelon Seeds from pumpkins Beans Tofu with Quinoa

Milk made from soy beans

BMI & Weight Management

If your goal for the low carb diet is to lose weight, you'll need to know your optimum body weight and how to interpret your present body weight. The Body Mass Index, or BMI calculation, is one of the most extensively used measures for determining your optimal weight.

BMI is calculated as follows:

1. Weigh yourself in pounds as a starting point.

2. Determine your height in inches.

3. Multiply the number of inches by the number of inches.

4. Multiply the result by your weight.

5. Multiply the result by 703 to get the total.

For example, if you are 60 inches tall and weigh 100 pounds, you should: 1.

$3600 = 60 \times 60$

$3..03 \times 703 = 21.09$ 2. $100 / 3600 = .03$

To calculate your BMI, use the table below:

Underweight is defined as a body mass index of 18.6 or below.

Ideal weight range: 18.7 to 24.8 lbs

Overweight is defined as having a body mass index of 24.9% to 29.9%.

Obesity is defined as a person who has reached the age of 30

Consult your doctor before beginning the low carb diet plan if your BMI indicates that you are underweight or obese. You could push your body to its limits if you stick to the diet and are underweight. Fat is designed to be utilized as an emergency fuel source for the body, particularly during sleep, so too much is just as dangerous as too little. If you're obese and you're on a diet, you'll need to keep track of how much weight you're losing. This is due to the possibility that your body may be unable to deal with the abrupt weight loss. When in doubt, seek expert assistance, particularly if your BMI falls between two extremes.

Because each individual is different, with their own health history and circumstances, weight reduction on the low carb diet will vary. Weight loss will be more substantial for certain people, particularly those who lead an active lifestyle, than for others who depend only on nutrition to lose weight.

This implies that you may not lose more than 7 pounds on this diet. However, one thing is certain: you will lose weight on this diet. Every pound lost should be used as incentive to keep the diet going. You may not achieve your target weight in a week, but with patience and dedication, you will achieve the weight you actually deserve.

Low-Carb Diet Types (Chapter 3)

The phrase "low carb diet" refers to a variety of diets that promote carb reduction in the pursuit of a better lifestyle and weight loss. While there are many different low carb diets, each with its own set of principles, regulations, and suggestions, they all have a low-carb foundation.

The following are some of the most well-known low-carb options:

1. Atkins

2. Stillman

3. Hollywood

4. Zone

5. Dukan

Diet: Atkins

Arguably the most popular low carb diet, the Atkins diet is the product of Dr. Robert Atkins. With an overweight condition himself, Atkins wanted to address and solve his weight problem. His weight loss method has been widely practiced and has provided various results.

The Atkins diet shares the same principles with the low carb diet because it significantly reduces the daily intake of carbs in meals. The low carb principles are translated into the four phases of the Atkins diet: induction, ongoing weight loss, pre-maintenance, and lifetime maintenance.

Induction is potentially the most difficult phase of the diet because it totally restricts followers from consuming any carb, or caps the intake to less than 20 grams a day. Within 2 weeks of this phase, the body consumes your fat content thereby reducing your weight. The next phase is the ongoing weight loss where the follower consumes incremental amounts of carbs until they reach their desired weight.

Once the weight is achieved, pre-maintenance phase follows, where the exact amount of carbs that do not allow weight gain is consumed. Once this quantity of carb is established, followers can start with the lifetime maintenance. This represents applying all the lessons learned from the previous phases, eating just enough carbs but still without gaining weight.

Stillman Diet

Named after its creator, Dr. Irwin Stillman, this diet is also low carb but not as restrictive as the Atkins diet. This diet actually came before the famous Atkins diet. Stillman was a doctor that specialized in obesity and he was regularly consulted by overweight patients.

Although it does not allow butter, dressings, fats or oils, this diet has no restrictions on consumption of lean beef, fish, poultry, eggs, spices, tea, and coffee. Preparation is also monitored; recipes are mostly baked, boiled, or broiled. Emphasis is also given on drinking 8 full

glasses of water and 7 small meals per day instead of a 3 large meals.

One criticism of the diet is that it does not allow enough fiber content in its recipes, resulting in an unbalanced diet. While it does offer weight reduction to more than 15 lbs in the first week of the diet alone, most followers need supplements of the nutrients they do not get from the limited food items.

Hollywood Diet

Named the Hollywood diet because it was created by Jamie Kabler, a popular nutritionist for Hollywood celebrities, this diet gained its reputation because of its promise of success within a short period of time. Instead of consuming low carb solid foods, this diet offers an orange- colored drink. This drink is a combination of various fruits' juice concentrates and is the only food source for at least 2 days.

After the consumption of this drink, the follower can undergo the Hollywood diet's 30-day miracle program. This program is meant to provide followers with the same weight loss benefits of the 2-day drink but this time with solid foods and with a meal that uses a Hollywood diet program product, such as the Mix Meal, the Meta Miracle, and other products.

Zone Diet

Aside from focusing on carbs alone, the Zone diet takes into consideration the role of insulin in weight. According to this diet, insulin, a hormone that balances blood sugar levels, is guilty for storing fat, which in turn increases weight. To control weight, the theory is you need to control your insulin levels. When dieters keep their insulin levels at the bare minimum, fat is burned and therefore more weight is lost.

This is where carbs come into the diet. When carbs are controlled, or also kept at a minimum but with an adequate consumption of protein and fats, insulin is controlled. This perfect balance of protein, fats, carbs, and insulin is referred to as the zone. This diet shows that followers can lose at least 5 pounds per week.

Dukan Diet

Although the Dukan diet has the same phases as with the Atkins diet, it is stricter. While the first phase of the Atkins allows a very minimal carb consumption, in the Dukan, even vegetables that are already low-carb are not allowed. Further restrictions include eggs, steaks, and pork chops.

The focus on this diet shifts to the importance of protein together with the elimination of carbs.

The idea behind the diet is that to maximize weight loss potential, aside from eliminating carbs, increased protein intake will reduce more weight. This is because the body requires more energy to break down and digest protein. At the same time, protein takes longer to digest and this allows the feeling of a full stomach to last longer. The result is that you burn more fats to digest proteins and you can also delay feelings of hunger longer than usual.

Servings: 4 Ingredients:

Part 2: The 7 Day Meal Plan Chapter 4: Ready, get set, lose! A burst of flavors to start your weight loss week Day One Meal Plan

Breakfast: Egg & Spinach Lunch: Coconut Beef Dinner: Chicken Skewers Snacks: Choco Mousse

Eggs & Spinach

Servings: 4 Ingredients:

4 eggs

10 oz. spinach

3 tbsp leek, chopped 1 tsp lemon juice

2 tbsp scallion, chopped 2 tbsp butter, divided\s1 clove garlic, halved 1 tsp

oregano, chopped\s1/4 tsp red pepper flakes 1/4 tsp paprika

2/3 cup plain Greek yogurt

2 tbsp olive oil

Salt and pepper Directions:\s1. Heat oven to 300 degrees

2. Put skillet on medium heat and add butter\s3. Add scallion and leek then set heat to low\s4. Cook for 10 minutes

5. Add lemon juice and spinach\s6. Add salt to taste\s7. Cook for another 5 minutes on high and turn the spinach until they

wilt

8. Transfer mixture to another skillet and make sure to leave liquid\s9. Use a spoon to make indentations on the mixture and crack the eggs into each indentation\s10. Bake for 15 minutes

11. Put saucepan on low heat and melt remaining butter 12. Sprinkle pepper flakes, paprika and salt and cook for another 2 minutes

13. Add oregano

14. Combine garlic, salt and yogurt in a bowl and set aside 15. Take garlic mixture and scoop garlic leaving only the yoghurt mixture

16. Spread mixture on top of baked eggs and drizzle with melted butter

17. Serve

Coconut Beef Servings: 4 Ingredients:

1 lb. steak, cut into thin strips

1 lb. pack of mixed stir fry vegetables 9 oz. rice noodles

3 tbsp red curry paste

4 tbsp coriander, chopped

2 tsp groundnut oil

9 oz. coconut milk 2 tbsp lime juice

1 tsp sugar Directions:\s1. Put together sugar, lime juice and paste with steak. Marinate for 5 minutes.

2. Place pan over medium heat and add marinated steak. Fry for 2 minutes.

3. Add milk and bring to a boil

4. Add vegetables and cook for another 5 minutes

5. Cook the noodles

6. Put noodles on bowl, top with the beef mixture

7. Top with coriander

8. Serve

Chicken Skewers

Servings: 3 Ingredients:

½ lb. chicken breast, cut into fillets

1 green pepper, remove the seeds 1 tbsp lemon juice

6 tbsp plain yogurt 2 tbsp curry paste

1 ripe mango, diced 1 tbsp lime juice

2 onions, chopped

Salt and pepper Directions: 1. Heat grill to medium for 15 minutes

2. Put together paste, lemon juice, yogurt and salt on shallow plate, mix well and set side

3. Cut the fillets into chunks and add into the yogurt mixture. Toss until the fillets are well coated.

4. Marinate the chicken for an hour while covered

5. Cut the pepper into squares. Skewer chicken and pepper in alternating order.

6. Put on grill and turn skewers to cook on all sides

7. Remove from grill when chicken is charred

8. Put together lime juice, onions and mango together, add salt and pepper to taste

9. Serve with mango salsa on the side

Choco Mousse Servings: 4 Ingredients:

1 1/2 cups heavy cream

6 packets Equal sugar substitute 1/2 teaspoon vanilla extract 1/4 cup

unsweetened cocoa powder

Directions:

1. Whip the cream with electric mixer.

2. Add Equal one packet at a time.

3. Add vanilla and cocoa powder, and beat until almost stiff.

4. Scrape down and mix again.

5. Place in serving dishes, cover, and refrigerate for at least 1/2 hour.

6. Serve within 4 hours of preparation.

Chapter 5: Here it comes! First pound down! Power meals without the guilt

Day Two Meal Plan

Breakfast: Pancakes Lunch: Roast Chicken Dinner: Salmon Frittatas Snacks:

Power Drink

Pancakes Servings: 2 Ingredient s: 1/2 cup besan flour 1 onion, chopped

1 tbsp olive oil

1/4 tsp garlic powder 1/4 tsp baking powder 1/2 cup water

Salt and pepper Direction: 1. Combine besan flour, baking powder, garlic powder, and salt and pepper in a bowl. Whisk together until completely mixed.

2. Add water and mix again, make sure there are no clumps

3. Put the vegetables in the mixture, set aside

4. Heat skillet to medium and add olive oil

5. Put the mixture and spread on the skillet. Cook each side for 5 minutes.

6. If desired, top with avocado, cashew, or other fruits and nuts 7. Serve

Roast Chicken

Servings: 4 Ingredients:

4 chicken breasts, skinned and deboned

1 onion, sliced 2 cloves garlic, diced 2 tbsp olive oil

1 cup tomatoes, diced

1 cup black olives, pitted and drained

½ tsp cumin

½ tsp paprika

½ tsp salt

½ tsp pepper Directions: 1. Heat oven to 350 degrees

2. Place pan over high heat and add olive oil

3. Add garlic and onion to pan and sauté for 2 minutes

4. Add olives, tomatoes, and chicken

5. Put together cumin, paprika, and salt and pepper in a small bowl and then sprinkle on top of chicken while cooking

6. Put pan inside oven and bake for 30 minutes

7. Serve

Salmon Frittatas Servings: 3 Ingredients:

2 oz. salmon, cut into ¼ inch pieces

3 eggs

4 egg whites

1 tbsp scallions, sliced into thin pieces 1/8 cup onion, diced ½ tbsp half and half 2 tbsp milk

2 oz. fat free cream cheese, cubed Salt and pepper

Directions:

1. Heat oven to 325 degrees

2. Place skillet on high heat and add oil

3. Sauté onions for 2 minutes 4. salt and pepper and then remove from heat 5. whites, half and half and milk in a bowl 6. cheese

7. with cooking spray 8. salmon mixture into ramekin 9. on top of salmon and fill until below the rim Add salmon and

Put eggs, egg Stir together with Spray ramekins Scoop 2 tbsp of

Pour egg mixture

10. Bake ramekins for 25 minutes

11. Serve

Power Drink Servings: 2 Ingredients:

1 avocado

½ cup Greek yogurt

1 tsp green tea powder

¼ cup protein powder, vanilla flavor

¼ cup almond milk, unsweetened 2 tsp sweetener

1 tbsp hot water Directions: 1. Mix together tea powder and hot water, set aside

2. Cut the avocado into chunks and put in blender

3. Add sweetener, yogurt, and protein powder into blender

4. Pour milk and tea mixture into blender

5. Blend into smooth consistency

6. Serve Servings: 4

Chapter 6: Keep it going, total lost- 2 to 3 pounds, reward yourself with these low-carb comfort foods

Day Three Meal Plan

Breakfast: Quinoa Bowl Lunch: Beef Stew Dinner: Buffalo Chicken Snacks: Crepes

Quinoa Bowl

Servings: 4 Ingredients:

4 eggs

1 cup quinoa

1 avocado, chopped 6 oz. salmon, smoked 2 tbsp olive oil

1 cup scallion, sliced 1 tbsp lemon juice

Salt and pepper Directions: 1. Cook quinoa, while it is cooking, heat skillet on medium

2. Cook eggs for 5 minutes, add salt and pepper to taste 3. Take the quinoa and layer with eggs first, then avocado, and then salmon cuts

4. Drizzle with the juice

5. Garnish with scallions

6. Serve

Beef Stew Servings: 4 Ingredients:

2 lbs. beef chuck roast, cut into cubes

8 0z tomato sauce

14.5 oz tomatoes with juice, diced 1 can low sodium beef broth

1 tbsp olive oil

1 cup cloves garlic, cut into slivers 2 tbsp capers

3 tbsp red wine vinegar 3 bay leaves

1 tsp oregano

1 cup olives cut into half

Salt and pepper Directions: 1. Add 1 tbsp of oil to pan over high heat

2. Cook beef cubes until they are brown on all sides

3. Put cubes in slow cooker and set aside

4. Pour broth into pan where cubes were cooked and simmer

5. Pour broth into slow cooker

6. Add remaining ingredients: olives, garlic, capers, oregano, tomatoes, vinegar, pepper, bay leaves and sauce into slow cooker

7. Set to high and cook for 4 hours

8. Serve

Buffalo Chicken Servings: 2 Ingredients:

5 chicken thighs, skinned

1 tsp seasoning

1/3 cup blue cheese 1 tbsp olive oil

1 tbsp Worcestershire sauce 1 tsp mustard

1 tsp hot sauce

½ tsp garlic powder

½ tsp onion powder 1 tbsp brown sugar

Salt and pepper Directions: 1. Heat oven to 400 degrees

2. Spray oil in baking dish

3. Trim the chicken of any fat and put in baking dish 4. Sprinkle seasoning, salt and pepper

5. Bake chicken for 15 minutes

6. Combine olive oil, Worcestershire sauce, mustard, sugar and onion and garlic powder together

7. Turn the chicken every 15 minutes, once turned glaze the sauce on each side. Repeat 3 times.

8. On the fourth time it is glazed, add the cheese on top and let it cook for another 10 minutes

9. Serve

Crepes Servings: 3 Ingredients: 2 eggs

2 egg whites

½ tsp baking soda

¼ cup coconut flour ¼ cup almond milk, unsweetened 2 tbsp flaxseed

Choice of berries Directions: 1. Heat skillet on high and coat with cooking spray

2. Mix all ingredients in a blender

3. Blend until completely combined

4. Pour mixture into skillet and completely cover it with the batter 5. Allow to cook until bubbles form and pop on top 6. After 3 minutes, flip crepe and cook the other side

7. Put berries inside the crepe and a few whole pieces on top 8.

Serve Servings: 12

Chapter 7: Halfway there, total pounds lost- 3 to 4! Classic meals with a low carb twist Day Four Meal Plan

Breakfast: Muffins Lunch: Meatballs Dinner: Tuna Patties Snacks: Berry Parfaits

Muffins

Servings: 12 Ingredients: 6 eggs

1 onion, thinly sliced

½ cup low fat cottage cheese

½ cup almond flour

½ cup parmesan cheese, grated

¼ cup flax seed

¼ cup yeast flakes

½ cup hemp seed Salt

Directions:

1. Heat oven to 375 degrees

2. Spray muffin pans with oil

3. In a large bowl, mix almond, cheese, flax seed, yeast flakes, baking

powder, hemp seed, and salt and set aside

4. In a separate bowl, mix eggs, cheese, and onions

5. Mix together powder mixture with egg mixture 6. Put combined mixture

into muffin cups

7. Bake for 30 minutes

8. Serve

Meatballs

Servings: 36 meatballs Ingredients:

1 lb lean ground beef

1 lb lean ground turkey

½ tsp allspice

½ tsp cardamom

¼ tsp cinnamon

¼ tsp white pepper

½ tsp ginger 1 tbsp garlic

1 onion

Salt Directions:

1. Heat oven to 400 degrees

2. Put both ground beef and turkey in a bowl and set aside

3. Slash onion and put in with meats, cinnamon, cardamom, garlic, ginger, salt and pepper, join thoroughly

4. Spray oil on barbecuing rack

5. Form balls by folding combination into your hands and spot them on grill

6. Bake for 30 minutes

7. Serve

Tuna Patties Servings: 1 Ingredients:

1 can of tuna, light 1

egg

¼ tsp garlic powder

1 tbsp onion, chopped

¼ tsp salt Directions: 1. Put skillet on medium hotness and splash with oil

2. Place all fixings in a bowl and blend together 3. Divide combination into 6 and scoop each into pan

4. Flatten in a size barely enough to flip with a spatula

5. Cook both sides

6. Serve

Berry Parfaits Servings: 3 Ingredients:

8 oz milk ricotta

1 tsp lemon zest

2 tbsp lemon juice

8 drops extract of stevia

1 cup of berries of choice Directions:

1. Put stevia, zing, juice, and ricotta in blender, blend for 2 minutes

2. Use clear glasses and make substitute layers of berries and ricotta mixture

3. Serve Servings: 4

Chapter 8: The goal is in sight! Full speed ahead with these easy recipes

Day Five Meal Plan

Breakfast: Breakfast Bake Lunch: White fish and capers Dinner: Chicken Pesto Snacks: Cookies

Breakfast Bake

Servings: 4 Ingredients: 12 turkey sausages

½ cup low fat mozzarella, grated 1 red bell pepper, chopped 1 green bell pepper, chopped 2 tsp olive oil

Pepper Directions: 1. Heat stove to 450 degrees

2. Cut red and green ringer peppers into 1 inch slices

3. Spray baking dish with oil and put peppers on the dish 4. Bake for 20 minutes

5. Put container on high hotness and add oil

6. Cook wieners for 10 minutes

7. Cut hotdogs into 1/3 size and add with the peppers in the oven 8. Bake for another 5 minutes

9. Take frankfurters from the broiler and sprinkle cheese 10. Put in broiler and set to broil 11. Broil for 2 minutes

12. Serve

White Fish and Capers

Servings: 3 Ingredients: 3 tilapia fillets

¼ cup parmesan cheddar, ground 2 tbsp olive oil 1 lemon

2 tbsp escapades and saline solution Salt and pepper Directions: 1. Place filets on a plate and shower 1 tbsp oil on all filets, both sides

2. Sprinkle salt and pepper on filets, set aside

3. Put cheddar in a wide bowl, set aside

4. Put dish on medium hotness and add 1 tbsp of oil

5. Dredge filets through cheddar and afterward put in pan 6. Cook each filet for 5 minutes on each side 7. Add tricks in container when time is nearly up

8. Squeeze lemon on fish 9. Serve

Chicken pesto

Servings: 3 Ingredients:

2 chicken breasts, skinned and deboned

1 onion

1 can chicken broth

½ can water 2 zucchini 1/3 cup pesto

2 tsp. all-purpose seasoning

1/3 cup vinaigrette dressing Salt and pepper

Directions:

1. Simmer stock and water in a saucepan

2. Add chicken and cook for 20 minutes

3. Remove chicken from stock and set aside

4. Mix together pesto, dressing, preparing, and pepper, set aside

5. Cut chicken and into cubes

6. Put chicken solid shapes and ¼ cup of pesto blend together in a container

7. Marinate for 1 hour

8. Slice onions and zucchini into flimsy cuts and put into bowl 9. Add remaining pesto sauce with the vegetables

10. Plate the chicken and serve

Cookies

Servings: 20 Ingredients:

1 egg

1 cup peanut butter 1

cup sweetener Directions:

1. Heat broiler to 350 degrees

2. Put all fixings in a bowl and blend together

3. Roll combination into 20 separate balls

4. Bake for 10 minutes

5. Serve Servings: 4

Chapter 9: Hang in there, easy recipes to get you going for the final push!

Day Six Meal Plan

Breakfast: Oatmeal

Lunch: Chinese Chicken Dinner: Mushroom Polenta Snacks: Ceviche

Oatmeal

Servings: 4 Ingredients: 2 tbsp cinnamon

½ cup unsweetened coconut, shredded into fine pieces

½ cup golden flax

½ cup chia seeds

2 tbsp unsweetened coconut milk

½ cup water Sweetener

Berries of choice Directions: 1. Mix flax, coconut, chia, and cinnamon

2. Scoop ½ cup of the combination and add water, put away for 5 minutes

3. Add milk and wanted measure of sugar and stir

4. Top with berries and serve

Chinese Chicken

Servings: 4 Ingredients:

Chicken ingredients

1 lb. chicken thighs, deboned and skinned

1/4 tsp garlic powder 1/4 tsp onion powder 1/8 cup soy sauce

1 tsp ginger

2 cups water Salad ingredients

1 cup cucumbers, sliced

1 cup Napa cabbage, shredded

1 cup white cabbage, shredded 1/4 cup scallions, sliced

1/8 cup cilantro, chopped 1 tbsp sesame seeds

1/4 cup radishes cut into thin slices Dressing ingredients

1/8 cup soy sauce

1/8 tsp Chinese mustard

1/2 tsp sesame oil

1/8 cup rice wine vinegar 1/2 tbsp sweetener

2 tbsp avocado oil 1/2 tbsp ginger paste

Directions: 1. Put chicken, garlic, onion powder, soy sauce, ginger, and water in pot. Bring to a boil.

2. Lower hotness and stew for 20 minutes

3. Remove chicken and shred, remove any remaining fat or tendons, set aside

4. Put the cabbages in a bowl and keep the middle piece void for the chicken

5. Add the cilantro, radishes, and scallions

6. Add the chicken in the middle 7. Sprinkle seeds on top and serve

Mushroom Polenta

Ingredients: Ingredients: Ingredients: Ingredients: Ingredients: ingredients: ingredients: ingredients:

8 mushroom caps that are flat

2 c. chevre

polenta (500 g) sliced Rocket leaves (50 g bag)

olive oil, 4 tbsp

75 grams chopped peppers

oregano, 2 tbsp

seasonings 1. Place mushrooms in a mixing bowl and drizzle with olive oil.

2. Preheat the grill to medium-high heat and cook the mushrooms for 5 minutes before removing from the grill.

3. Add the peppers and oregano.

4. Finish with the cheese.

5. Re-ignite the grill and wait for the cheese to melt.

6. Grill the polenta for 5 minutes on each side. 7. Arrange the rocket leaves on top of the polenta.

8. Season to taste with salt and pepper 9. Put out the food

3 Ceviche Servings

8 oz. sliced button mushrooms

12 ounces vegetable stock a third of a lemon

12 sliced red bell pepper

12 sliced green bell pepper 1 chopped onion

garlic, 2 cloves

1 tblsp chopped cilantro

honey (14 tsp)

1 teaspoon chopped jalapeno

1 teaspoon of extra virgin olive oil

seasonings 1. In a skillet, cook garlic for 2 minutes on medium heat.

2. Mash garlic and add to a bowl with onion, red and green peppers, and mushrooms; set aside. 3. In a separate bowl, combine all fixings and mix well.

4. Add the mushroom mixture to the preparedness.

5. Refrigerate overnight in a covered container.

6. Serve 2 people

Chapter 10: 6–7 pounds lost! Congratulations!

Meal Plan For Day 7

Veggie Hash (breakfast) Meatloaf (lunch) Shrimp Salad for Dinner Pepper Poppers are a delicious snack to have on hand.

Hash of veg

Ingredients: Ingredients: Ingredients: Ingredients: Ingredients: Ingredients: Ingredients

34 pound cauliflower, diced

1 onion

olive oil, 2 tbsp

1 garlic clove (chopped) lemon juice, 2 tblsp

paprika (14 tbsp) water, 3 tbsp

seasonings 1. Heat the oil in a skillet over high heat. 2. Add the onion and cauliflower and cook for 3 minutes, stirring occasionally.

3. Combine the paprika, salt, pepper, and water in a large mixing bowl.

4. Cook for another 5 minutes covered in skillet.

5. Reduce the heat to low and stir in the garlic for another 2 minutes.

6. Cook for 30 seconds after adding the lemon juice. 7. Put out the food

4 servings of meatloaf

1 pound grass-fed ground beef

eggs (three)

shredded cheese, 1/2 cup 4 ounces diced green pepper sour cream, 1/8 cup

a garlic clove cumin (1/4 teaspoon)

chili powder (1/2 teaspoon) 1. Preheat the oven to 400 degrees Fahrenheit and preheat the broiler.

2. In a separate bowl, whisk together the eggs and set them aside.

3. Combine the hamburger, eggs, cumin, and stew powder in a large mixing bowl. 4. Roll the hamburger mixture halfway on waxed paper to create a level square.

5. Arrange half of the bean stew on top, then sprinkle with cheddar.

6. Continue rolling the other side into a loaf.

7. Peel the wax paper away.

8. Fold the portion closures to keep the stew and cheddar from spilling.

9. Place a portion of the stew in a dish and top with the remaining stew, cheddar, and cream.

10. Cook for 1 hour.

11. Serve

Salad with salmon and shrimp

Ingredients: 1 serving

100 g cooked salmon, cut into bite-sized pieces

1 quart of spinach

1 watercress cup

Cooked prawns (10 prawns) Greek yogurt 100 g 2 tablespoons dill

1 tablespoon lemon juice

a wedge of lemon 1. In a mixing bowl, combine yogurt, zing from lemon wedge, dill, and pepper; mix well and set aside.

2. Toss the vegetables with the salmon in a bowl.

3. Top with prawns and a dollop of yogurt dressing.

Poppers made with peppers

Ingredients: 4 servings

12 pound peppers, baby

4 oz chopped and cooked bacon 1 teaspoon of hot sauce

2 tablespoons cilantro, chopped

1 tbsp lime juice Salt

Directions:

1. Preheat the oven to 350°F.

2. Remove the peppers' stems and cut them lengthwise. 3. Remove the seeds and membrane.

4. Bake peppers for 10 minutes on a baking sheet.

5. Mash avocados and combine with hot sauce, cilantro, and lime juice in a mixing bowl.

6. Season with salt and pepper to taste. 7. Scoop guacamole into the pepper's empty piece.

8. Toss with bacon and serve. Serves 8 people

More Low-Carb/High-Fat Recipes in Chapter 11

Breakfast Dishes 8 servings Hashbrown Potato Cakes Ingredients:

1 pound red potatoes (round or russet)

1 medium onion, thinly sliced 1 tablespoon of extra virgin olive oil

2 teaspoons fresh thyme snipped or 1/4 teaspoon crushed dried thyme a quarter teaspoon salt

1/8 teaspoon black pepper, freshly ground

Directions for nonstick cooking spray:

1. Preheat the oven to 300°F.

2. Peel and coarsely shred potatoes, then rinse in a colander with cold water.

3. Drain well, squeezing delicately, then wipe off with paper towels and place in a large bowl. The onion slices should be quartered. Toss the potatoes with the onion, oil, thyme, salt, and pepper.

4. Lightly spray a nonstick skillet or frying pan that hasn't been heated with nonstick cooking spray.

5. Heat a skillet or cast iron pan over medium heat.

6. Scoop a slightly adjusted estimating tablespoon of the potato mixture onto a skillet or griddle for each cake.

7. Using a spatula, evenly straighten the potato blend. Cook for 5 minutes before serving. Turn potato cakes carefully with a wide spatula (be careful not to turn them too soon or they will fall apart). 8. Cook for an additional 3 to 5 minutes, or until golden brown.

9. Arrange the cooked potato cakes on a cookie sheet.

10. Keep warm in the broiler, uncovered, while you finish the rest of the potato cakes.

11. Repeat with the outstanding potato blend, frequently mixing the two together.

Pizza Waffles with Low Carbs

Ingredients: 5 servings

5 separate eggs

4 tbsp coconut flour, salt and pepper to taste

1 tbsp. dried spices (I use rosemary and oregano) 1 teaspoon of baking powder 1 stick 125g/4.5oz + 1 tbs softened margarine 3 tbsp. whole milk

12 c. grated cheese

1. Whip the egg whites until they are firm and have hardened peaks.

2. Combine the egg yolks, coconut flour, salt, spices, and baking powder in a separate bowl.

3. Gradually drizzle in the liquefied spread, blending to ensure a smooth consistency.

4. Combine the milk and ground cheddar cheese in a mixing bowl. Blend everything together thoroughly.

5. Gently fold spoonfuls of whisked egg whites into the yolk mixture. Attempt to retain as much air and volume as possible.

6. Pour enough waffle batter into the warm waffle maker to make one waffle. Cook until golden brown on both sides.

7. Continue until the entire blend has been used.

Salad with Low Carb Eggs

Serves 6 hard-boiled eggs

12 cup mayonnaise, full fat 12 – 1 teaspoon curry powder (to taste)

1. Place the eggs in a pan and cover them with COLD water to make the bubbled eggs.

2. Turn on the heat and wait for the water to bubble for 7 minutes.

3. Drain and rinse with cold water to keep them from overcooking.

4. Once the eggs have cooled, peel them and chop them into small pieces.

5. Combine the eggs, mayonnaise, and curry powder in a bowl.

6. Garnish with cleaved fresh parsley.

Tacos de Breakfast

2 tacos 22 eggs

1/8 teaspoon oregano 1 gram oregano 1/8 teaspoon cumin, 1 gram cumin a pinch of salt and pepper 22 tortillas with a low carb count

2 tblsp

Avocado (18.75 g) 2 tblsp 1 tablespoon salsa

1. Lightly coat a microwave-safe dish in cooking spray.

2. Combine the eggs, cumin, oregano, salt, and pepper in a mixing bowl. If you're adding more vegetables, toss them in as well. If your vegetables aren't quite ready, microwave them for 1-2 minutes until just tender.

3. Cook the eggs for one minute in the microwave. Remove and scramble with a fork. Return to the microwave for another 1-1.5 minutes, or until thoroughly cooked.

4. Heat the tortillas for 10-15 seconds in the microwave.

5. Fill your tacos with your favorite salsa, avocado, and any additional toppings.

Scones with Cinnamon Rolls (serves 4) Ingredients: 8 Scones:

2 CUP ALMONDFUL

3 tbsp Swerve 2 tablespoons baking powder

1/2 teaspoon salt

1/4 teaspoon cinnamon powder 1 large, lightly beaten egg

melted 1/4 cup coconut oil 2 tbsp cream

1 tsp vanilla 3 tbsp Swerve Sweetener

2 teaspoons cinnamon Icing:

Directions: 1 oz. cream cheddar scones, relaxed 1 tablespoon of cream 1/2 tbsp softened spread

1 tbsp powdered sugar Swerve is a natural sweetener that comes in a variety of flavors. a quarter teaspoon vanilla extract

1. Preheat the oven to 325 degrees Fahrenheit and line a baking sheet with parchment paper. In a large mixing bowl, whisk together almond flour, sugar,

baking powder, salt, and cinnamon. Combine the egg, coconut oil, cream, and vanilla extract in a mixing bowl until the batter comes together.

2. Icing Whisk together the filling ingredients in a small mixing bowl. Half of the filling should be sprinkled into the batter and blended in, but not completely combined, in order to keep the filling streaky.

3. Pour the mixture onto a parchment-lined baking sheet and pat it into a rough circle about 7 or 8 crawls across. Finish with a sprinkling of besting. Cut into 8 even wedges, carefully separate them, and place them evenly on the baking sheet. Prepare the scones for 20 to 25 minutes, or until firm and lightly seared. Keep an eye on the bottoms to make sure they don't burn.

4. Remove the pan from the heat and place it on a wire rack to cool.

1. Cream together cream cheddar, margarine, and cream until smooth.

2. Mix in powdered sugar and vanilla extract until smooth.

3. Using a pastry bag, pipe or spread the mixture over the cooled scones.

Pancakes with lemon ricotta

Syrup of Mixed Berries:

1 cup frozen berries (mixed)

2 tbsp sugar = 1/4 cup water xanthan gum (quarter teaspoon)

Pancakes: Syrup:

a third of a cup of ricotta 3 huge eggs

lemon juice, 1/4 cup 1 lemon zest 1/4 cup water

1 pound almond flour

a sweetener equivalent to 1/4 cup sugar 2 tbsp flour de coco (coconut flour)

1 1/2 teaspoons of baking powder 1/4 teaspoon salt For the pan, use either butter or oil.

1. Combine the berries, water, and sweetener in a medium pan over medium heat.

2. Bring to a boil, then reduce heat and simmer until berries are tender enough to crush with a fork.

3. Add the thickener and whisk vigorously to combine. Set aside to thicken.

Pancakes:

1. Combine the ricotta, eggs, lemon juice, water, and lemon zing in a blender. Mix for about 10 seconds, or until everything is evenly blended.

2. Combine almond flour, sugar, coconut flour, baking powder, and salt in a mixing bowl until smooth.

3. Add spread or oil to a frying pan or large skillet and heat over medium heat. When the skillet is hot, spoon about 3 tbsp of player into 4 inch circles and cook until the edges are dry, there are a couple of little air pockets on top, and the underside is a brilliant brown. Cook until the second side is a brilliant brown, about 2 to 3 minutes.

4. Remove the hotcakes from the pan and keep them warm while rehashing with the leftover batter. You should be able to get about 12 pancakes out of this recipe.

5. Top hotcakes with berry syrup and spread.

Lunchtime Dishes Pasta with Broccoli Slaw (Serves 4) Ingredients: 2

1 12-ounce bag of dry broccoli slaw (4 cups)

1 cup low-fat smooth tomato soup (like Amy's Chunky Tomato Bisque) or squashed tomatoes from the can

1 teaspoon hacked garlic (or more, according to preference) a dash of onion powder or more, to taste a dash of salt and dark pepper, to taste a dash of squashed red pepper, to taste

3 tbsp reduced fat parmesan-style ground beef, divided

1. Preheat a nonstick skillet to medium-high heat on the stove.

2. Stir in 1/4 cup water and the slaw. Cook, stirring occasionally, until the water has evaporated and the slaw has relaxed slightly, about 5 to 8 minutes.

3. Stir in the soup/tomatoes, garlic, seasonings, and 2 tablespoons ground beef. Cook, stirring occasionally, until the mixture is hot, about 3 to 4 minutes.

4. Season to taste with additional flavors if desired. Top with staying 1 tablespoon ground besting. Enjoy!

Honey Soy Broiled Salmon

Ingredients:\sDirections:

1 scallion, minced

2 tablespoons decreased sodium soy sauce 1 tablespoon rice vinegar

1 tablespoon honey

1 teaspoon minced new ginger

1 pound place cut salmon filet, cleaned (see Tip) and cut into 4 portions 1 teaspoon toasted sesame seeds,

Tips:

1. Whisk scallion, soy sauce, vinegar, honey and ginger in a medium bowl until the honey is broken up. Place salmon in a sealable plastic bag,

2. Add 3 tablespoons of the sauce and refrigerate; let marinate for 15 minutes. Save the excess sauce.

3. Preheat oven. Line a little baking dish with foil and coat with cooking spray.

4. Transfer the salmon to the skillet, cleaned side down. (Dispose of the marinade.) Broil the salmon 4 to 6 crawls from the hotness source until cooked through, 6 to 10 minutes. Sprinkle with the held sauce and trimming with sesame seeds.

How to skin a salmon filet: Place skin-side down. Beginning at the last part, slip a long blade between the fish tissue and the skin, holding down solidly with your other hand. Tenderly push the sharp edge along at a 30° point, isolating the filet from the skin without slicing through either.

To toast sesame seeds, heat a little dry skillet over low hotness. Add seeds and mix continually, until brilliant and fragrant, around 2 minutes. Move to a little bowl and let cool.

People with celiac illness or gluten-affectability should utilize soy sauces that are named"sans gluten," as soy sauce might contain wheat or other glutencontaining sugars and flavors.

Chicken and Asparagus Stir fry

Serves 4\sIngredients:

Directions:

1 1/2 pounds skinless chicken bosom, cut into 1-inch solid shapes Kosher salt, to taste 1/2 cup decreased sodium chicken broth 2 tablespoons diminished sodium shoyu or soy sauce (or Tamari for GF) 2 teaspoons cornstarch

2 tablespoons water

1 tbsp canola or grapeseed oil, divided

1 pack asparagus, closes managed, cut into 2-inch pieces 6 cloves garlic, chopped 1 tbsp new ginger

3 tablespoons new lemon squeeze new dark pepper, to taste

1. Lightly prepare the chicken with salt. In a little bowl, join chicken stock and soy sauce. In a

subsequent little bowl join the cornstarch and water and blend well to combine.

2. Heat a large non-stick wok over medium-high heat, when hot add 1 teaspoon of the oil, then add the asparagus and cook until tender-crisp, about 3 to 4 minutes. Add the garlic and ginger and cook until brilliant, around 1 moment. Set aside.

3. Increase the heat to high, then add 1 teaspoon of oil and half of the chicken and cook until browned and cooked through, about 4 minutes on each side. Eliminate and put away and rehash with the excess oil and chicken. Set aside.

4. Add the soy sauce combination; heat to the point of boiling and cook around 1-1/2 minutes. Add lemon juice and cornstarch combination and mix well, when it stews return the chicken and asparagus to the wok and blend well, eliminate from heat and serve.

5. Heat a large non-stick wok over medium-high heat, when hot add 1 teaspoon of the oil, then add the asparagus and cook until tendercrisp, about 3 to 4 minutes. Add the garlic and ginger and cook until brilliant, around 1 moment. Set aside.

6. Increase the heat to high, then add 1 teaspoon of oil and half of the chicken and cook until browned and cooked through, about 4 minutes on each side. Eliminate and put away and rehash with the excess oil and chicken. Set aside.

7. Add the soy sauce combination; heat to the point of boiling and cook around 1-1/2 minutes. Add lemon juice and cornstarch combination and mix well, when it stews return the chicken and asparagus to the wok and blend well, eliminate from heat and serve.

Shawarma Chicken Bowls with Basil-Lemon Vinaigrette

Serves 4 Ingredients: Chicken Shawarma

1 lb / 453 gr free-range organic chicken breast, cut into 3-inch strips

2 tablespoons olive oil

2 tablespoons lemon juice

¾ teaspoon fine grain sea salt 3 garlic cloves, minced

1 teaspoon curry powder

½ teaspoon ground cumin

¼ teaspoon ground coriander

Salad

6 cups / 3.5 oz / 100 gr spring greens

1 cup / 5.3 oz / 150 gr cherry tomatoes, halved 2 handfuls torn fresh basil leaves 1 avocado, sliced

Basil-Lemon Vinaigrette

2 large handfuls fresh basil leaves 1

clove garlic, smashed

½ teaspoon fine grain sea salt

2 tablespoons fresh lemon juice 5 tablespoons olive oil

6 cups / 3.5 oz / 100 gr spring greens

1 cup / 5.3 oz / 150 gr cherry tomatoes, halved 2 handfuls torn fresh basil leaves

1 avocado, sliced Directions:\s1. In a bowl whisk olive oil, lemon juice, garlic, salt, curry powder, cumin and coriander until combined.

2. In a shallow sealable holder or in a huge Ziploc sack, consolidate chicken tenders and marinade.

3. Cover or seal and marinate in the cooler for no less than 20 minutes (marinate for the time being for fullest flavor.)

4. When you're prepared to make the dinner, heat a huge nonstick skillet over medium-high heat.

5. Add a smidgen of olive oil, add the chicken and cook until brilliant brown and cooked through, around 6 to 8 minutes turning routinely, until juices run clear.

6. Meanwhile make the vinaigrette. In a food processor (or little blender), process the basil, garlic, salt, and lemon juice until smooth. With the engine running, gradually add the oil. Mix until consolidated. Set aside.

7. To make the plates of mixed greens, add the greens in an enormous bowl and throw them with a sprinkle of salt and pepper. Add the chicken on top alongside the tomatoes, basil, and avocado.

8. Drizzle the bowl with the basil-lemon vinaigrette and serve.

Spaghetti Squash Noodle Bowl with Lime Peanut Sauce Serves 4

Ingredients: Squash noodle

1 large spaghetti squash, cut in half lengthwise + seeds scooped out 4 kale stalks, stems removed 1 shallot, peeled

1/2 cup chopped toasted nuts of your preference (cashews) 3 tbsp sesame seeds (toasted, raw)

chopped leafy herb if you like (cilantro, mint, thai basil etc) 1 bunch of broccoli, cut into florets salt + pepper

Lime peanut sauce

1/2 inch fresh ginger, peeled + rough chopped 2

peeled garlic cloves + coarsely chopped

1-2 tablespoons sriracha (or other hot sauce you like)

peanut butter, 2 tbsp (or tahini, sunflower seed butter, almond butter etc)

1 lime, peeled and diced 1 tbsp vinegar (rice)

2 tablespoons agave nectar

1 tbsp soy sauce (tamari)

extra virgin coconut oil, a little spoonful (optional) 1/4 teaspoon sesame oil, roasted

a half-cup of grapeseed oil 1. Preheat the oven to 375 degrees Fahrenheit.

2. Place the squash halves, cut side down, on a baking sheet lined with material. Heat for approximately an hour, or until the tissue begins to peel away in strands.

3. While the squash cooks, cut the kale leaves into 1/3-inch strips and place them in a large mixing bowl. Cut the shallot in half lengthwise, then cut the halves into thin half-moons and store. Remove the spices and roasted nuts from the shallows and set them aside.

4. Once the broccoli has been sliced, heat a medium saucepan with about an inch of water over medium heat. Toss it into a stew. Place the broccoli florets in a liner container and keep them in the refrigerator until just before serving.

5. In a blender, combine all of the sauce ingredients and process until smooth. Set aside after tasting for preparation.

6. When the squash is cold enough to handle, add the broccoli liner container to the stewing water in the saucepan. Cover and steam broccoli for 3-4 minutes, or until desired doneness is reached. Scratch the spaghetti threads

out with a fork into the large basin with the sliced greens while the broccoli is steaming. The heat from the squash should slightly shrink the greens. Pour a generous amount of dressing into the bowl, season with salt and pepper, and toss the squash and kale gently.

7. Remove the broccoli from the heat source. Divide the squash and kale into four separate bowls. Add steamed broccoli, chopped shallots, slashed almonds, sesame seeds, hacked spices, and additional sauce to each dish.

Recipes for Dinner Cheeseburger Casserole feeds 6 people.

Ingredients: Casserole

2 lbs lean ground sirloin 5 slices bacon, chopped a quarter teaspoon of chili powder

a quarter teaspoon of garlic powder

12 tsp. salt 14 tsp. pepper a single egg

8 oz. Italian cheddar blend (or cheddar or your favorite)

1. Preheat the oven to 350 degrees Fahrenheit.

2. Place the bacon in a pan and cook for 5-7 minutes over medium heat.

3. Toss in the ground hamburger and heat until both sides are browned.

4. Add stew powder, garlic powder, salt, and pepper to taste.

5. Stir in the egg and half of the cheese.

6. Place the beef mixture in a greased 2-quart goulash dish.

7. Finish with the remaining cheese.

8. Bake for 35 minutes, uncovered, until hot and bubbling.

9. Garnish with garnishes of your choosing and serve.

Garnish 2 cups shredded lettuce 1 gallon sour cream

a quarter cup of spicy sauce

Lamb Chops with a Low-Carb Herb Crusade

Ingredients: 2 large garlic cloves, smashed, or 112 tablespoons bumped garlic 1 fresh thyme branch, cut

1 rosemary twig, freshly trimmed 1 teaspoon salt (fit)

1 tbsp extra-virgin extra-virgin olive oil 4 114-inch cuts in the sheep's midsection

1. Crush the garlic cloves and cut the spices into small pieces (leave the stems behind first). In a large mixing basin, combine them with the salt and a substantial quantity of the olive oil. Add the sheep cleaves and cover them with them. Place the bowl in the refrigerator and set aside for 30 minutes to marinate. Alternatively, do this a couple of hours ahead of time to get a head start on supper.

2. Preheat the broiler to 400 degrees F about 25 minutes before serving. Pour the remaining olive oil into a pan with a heat-resistant handle and a high heat setting. Add the slashes on both sides and earthy color them for about 3 minutes each.

3. Place a plate on the heat and cook the sheep hacks until they're cooked to your liking. Around 10 minutes is considered somewhat unusual. Place them on serving dishes after they're done.

Allow 5 minutes for resting before serving.

Roasted Barramundi with Tomato and Olive Relish serves 6 to 8 people.

2\sIngredients: Directions:

2 fillets 5-6 oz. Barramundi (or equivalent delicate white fish) per 2 tsp. olive oil for scrubbing fish

Szeged Fish Rub, 2 tsp., for scrubbing fish 1/4 cup cherry tomatoes, finely chopped 1/4 cup dark olives, thinly sliced

1/4 cup green olives, finely chopped 1 teaspoon lemon zest

2 t lemon juice, freshly squeezed (zing the lemon first, and afterward crush the juice) 2 t new parsley, finely cut 1 tablespoon olive oil, freshly ground dark pepper to taste

1. Defrost the fish for a few hours or overnight in the refrigerator. If your filets have an afterthought fold of incredibly delicate fish, clip it off since it will be overdone when the thicker sections are done.

2. Preheat the broiler or toaster to 400 degrees Fahrenheit/200 degrees Celsius. Rub the fish on both sides with olive oil and a generous amount of Szeged Fish Rub, rubbing it into the flesh. Place the fish on a boiling sheet. While the broiler heats up, let the fish to come to room temperature while you prepare the relish.

3. Chop the cherry tomatoes, dark olives, and green olives into small pieces. After squeezing the lemon and crushing the juice, measure out 2 teaspoons lemon juice. (If you have any leftover lemon juice, just put it in the freezer.) 2 tablespoons level or wavy parsley, chopped Combine the tomatoes, black olives, green olives, lemon zest, lemon juice, and olive oil in a mixing bowl, and season with a pinch of salt and freshly crushed dark pepper.

4. Place the fish in the broiler or toaster when it's room temperature, and cook for 10-12 minutes, or until it's just firm to the touch. Serve immediately with a generous spoonful of the tomato and olive relish.

Italian Shrimp with Low Carbohydrates (Serves 4) 1\sIngredients: Directions:

2 tablespoons olive oil 1 garlic clove, chopped

a quarter teaspoon of salt

12 tblsp oregano

1 pound cooked medium shrimp from Daily ChefTM 14 cup Signature Italian Dressing from Olive Garden

1. Follow the thawing instructions on the pack.

2. Preheat the sauté container to medium heat. Pour olive oil into the pan.

3. Toss in the garlic and shrimp. Assemble the shrimp on the pan in an equal layer.

4. Stir the shrimp and re-orchestrate them, being sure to cook all sides. Remove the mixture from the pan after it has become delicate and softly crisped, about 2-5 minutes.

5. Toss the shrimp with the Olive Garden dressing and other seasonings. With aspects that are desired.

Chicken Cooked in the Oven

1/3 cup low-fat buttermilk (optional)

1/4 cup finely hacked new chives 1 teaspoon mustard (Dijon) a quarter teaspoon of spicy sauce

4 chicken bosoms (bone-in) 1/2 cup breadcrumbs (dry) a half teaspoon of salt

1/2 teaspoon pepper, freshly ground

1. Combine the buttermilk, chives, mustard, and spicy sauce in a medium mixing basin. Remove the skin from the chicken bosoms, place the chicken in a mixing basin, and let it soak for 30 minutes or overnight.

2. Preheat the oven to 425 degrees Fahrenheit. Using a cooking spray, spray a rimmed baking sheet. In a broad, shallow basin, place the breadcrumbs.

3. Season the chicken with salt and pepper after removing it from the marinade.

4. Toss the chicken in the breadcrumbs to thoroughly coat it. Place the chicken on a baking sheet that has been prepared ahead of time.

5. Spray the chicken well with cooking spray and cook for 25 to 30 minutes, or until it is just cooked through.

Recipes for Snacks Skillet Pizza (Serves 1)

Handful of crumbled mozzarella cheddar - just enough to fill the bottom half of a 10-inch pan

1-2 tablespoons squished tomatoes (canned) (no sugar added) Slices of pepperoni powdered garlic

dried basil or Italian seasoning

New basil, crushed red pepper, and Parmesan cheddar (optional)

1. Preheat a small nonstick skillet over medium heat.

2. Evenly cover the bottom half of the heated skillet with crumbled mozzarella cheese.

3. Using the back of a spoon, lightly sprinkle the smashed tomatoes on top of the cheddar, leaving a border around the borders of the cheese crust.

4. Add garlic powder, dried basil, or Italian seasoning to taste. Arrange the pepperoni on top.

5. Cook until the mixture is sizzling, foaming, and the edges are brown. With a spatula, try to raise up the pizza's edges. It will easily pull up from the skillet after it has finished cooking. If this is the case,

When something sticks, it's a sign that it's not quite ready. Continue to elevate and check often. Work spatula softly and progressively beneath to relax entire pizza and transfer to a cutting board when it finally starts to pull up effectively without sticking.

6. If preferred, garnish with Parmesan, fresh torn basil leaves, and smashed red pepper.

7. Set aside for 5 minutes to cool. While it cools, the exterior will firm much more.

Cut into pizza shapes using a pizza shaper, transfer to a serving platter, and enjoy!

Ingredients for Pepperoni Chips: 1 box (normal or turkey) pepperonis

Directions:

1. Place two paper towels on top of each other and add as many pepperonis as desired, making sure they don't overlap. Using an additional paper towel, cover the dish.

2. Microwave the pepperonis for about 1 minute, or until they are stiffened and solid.

3. If you want more pepperoni crisps, repeat the process. Serve with a low-carb plunge or, my personal favorite, salsa!

Ingredients for Zucchini Pizza:

Directions:

1 zucchini, cleaned well and with the ends chopped off

a quarter-cup of spaghetti sauce

1 cup crumbled mozzarella

1. Preheat the oven to 350 degrees Fahrenheit.

2. Spritz with frying splash (or gently wipe olive oil on baking sheet).

3. Cut zucchini into 14-inch slices and place on baking pan.

4. Drizzle sauce over the pieces.

5. Top with mozzarella, cheddar, and any additional toppings you choose.

6. Bake until the cheddar has melted and become a magnificent brown color, then remove and cool.

7. Enjoy!

Cheesy Egg Chips with Zero Carbs

Ingredients: 4 Egg Whites (serves 1)

2 tbsp shredded cheddar in the flavor of your choice salt and pepper to taste if required 1/2 tbsp water to thin it down a bit

1. Preheat the broiler to 400°F and grease a medium nonstick biscuit pan.

2. Whisk together your egg whites, water, and any seasonings you'll be using.

3. Using a needle, dispense about 2.5ml of the egg white mixture into each biscuit cup, just enough to cover the bottom.

4. Toss a smidgeon of the desired cheddar onto each egg white.

5. Bake for 15 minutes to get a good mash without replicating, but check them after a few minutes to make sure they're done.

6. Once they've reached your preferred crunch, remove them from the burner and enjoy them with any low-carb dip or on their own.

8 servings cheesy cauliflower breadsticks Ingredients: 4 cups riced cauliflower (around 1 enormous head of cauliflower)

4 eggs • 2 cups mozzarella cheese • 3 tablespoons oregano • 4 garlic cloves, chopped • salt and pepper to taste • 1 to 2 cups mozzarella cheddar (for topping)

1. Preheat the broiler to 425 degrees Fahrenheit. Prepare two pizza plates or a large baking sheet lined with parchment paper.

2. Check to see whether your cauliflower florets are typically cut. In a food processor, pulse the cauliflower florets until they resemble rice.

3. Cover the cauliflower with the top of a microwavable holder. 10 minutes in the microwave In a large mixing bowl, combine the microwaved cauliflower, 4 eggs, 2 cups mozzarella, oregano, garlic, and salt and pepper. Combine everything in a blender.

4. Divide the mixture in half and place each half on the prepared baking sheets, shaping either a pizza outer layer or a rectangle shape for the breadsticks.

5. Bake for about 25 minutes, or until the hull is extremely golden (no garnish yet). Try not to be concerned about the fact that the exterior isn't drenched in any manner. Sprinkle with exceptional mozzarella cheddar and return to the burner for another 5 minutes, or until the cheddar has melted.

6. Cut into slices and serve.

Conclusion

I'm certain that after reading this book, you've worked out how to practice the low-carb, high-protein diet on your own. Remember your low-carbohydrate, high-protein diet; you'll appreciate this summary on your next trip to the supermarket. You may concentrate on your optimum body weight by recording your BMI and comparing it to the recommended reaches.

I am certain that you will be able to start your low carb diet lifestyle by following the suggested guidelines in this book. Keep in mind that these are only a few of the various layouts available, as well as the ones that you may develop yourself. Use your imagination when it comes to the low carb and high protein dietary categories; this way, you'll be able to enjoy the tastes you want while losing the weight you don't want.

After you've finished reading this book, you should go to your storeroom or kitchen. Start stocking up on low-carb and high-protein food ingredients to employ in your diet. Simultaneously, eliminate non-low carb diet cordial ingredients, since this will remove the allure of using them. Consider bringing home-cooked meals to your place of business. The great majority of the food supplied in your cafeteria may not meet your diet's low carb requirements.

Start backing out of your usual carb stacking a few days before you start the eating regimen. When making a request, ask for lean meat and avoid high-carbohydrate snacks at work. This manner, you'll be more than ready when you start the entire eating regimen on Day 1. This will prevent crashes, which are common among those who begin an eating regimen unprepared.

Your dream of achieving your ideal weight might become a reality thanks to the low carb and high protein diet! Begin practicing the low-carb diet way of life and preparing low-carb meals right now!

Last Thoughts...

Thank you very much for taking the time to download this book!

Finally, assuming you found this book to be worthwhile, if it isn't too much bother, set aside some time to express your thoughts and write a review.

Thank you for your time and consideration, and best wishes!

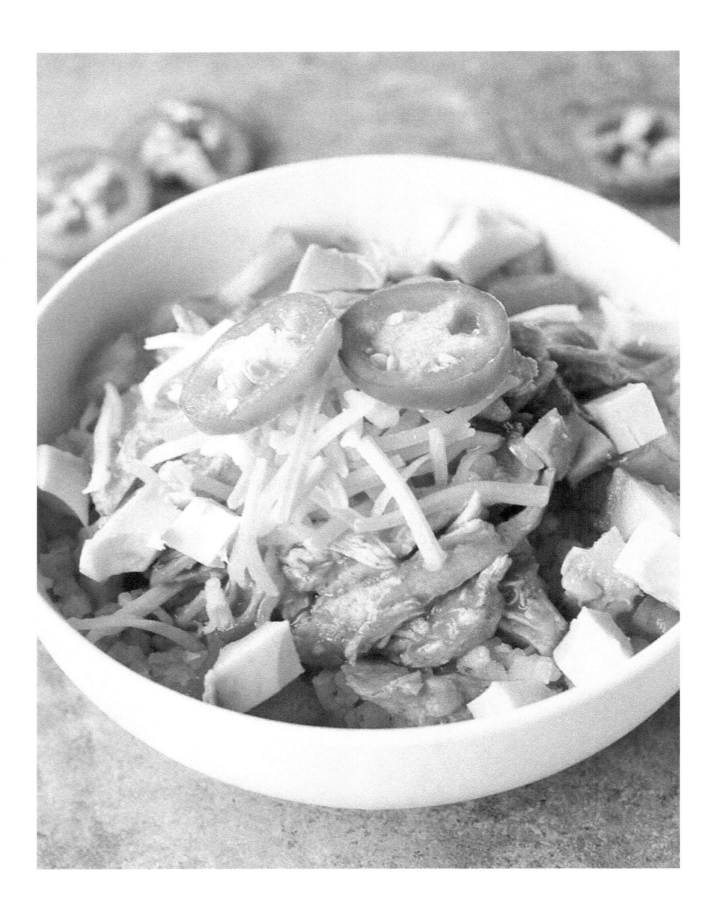

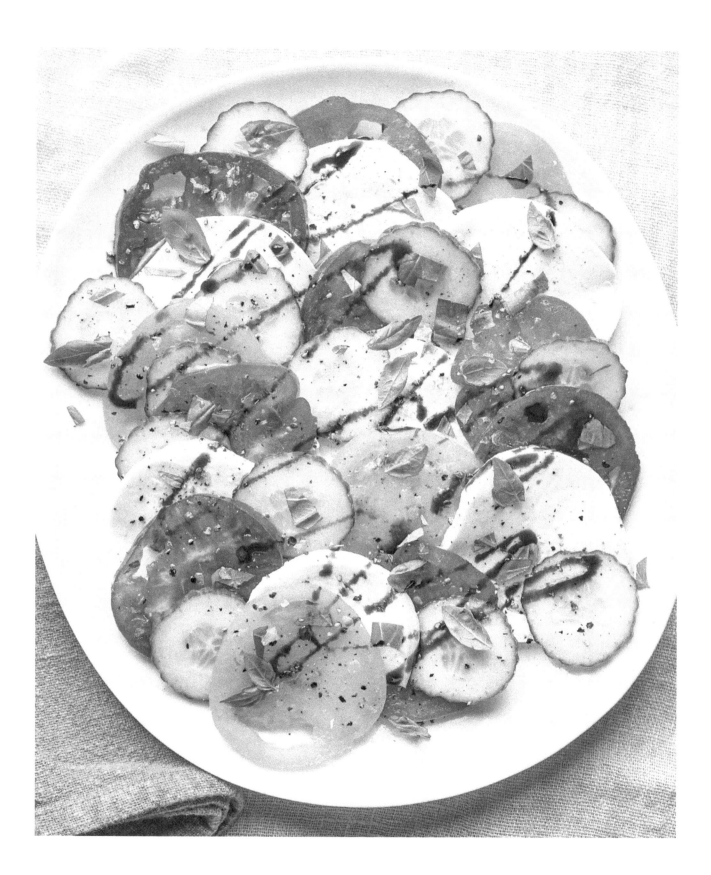

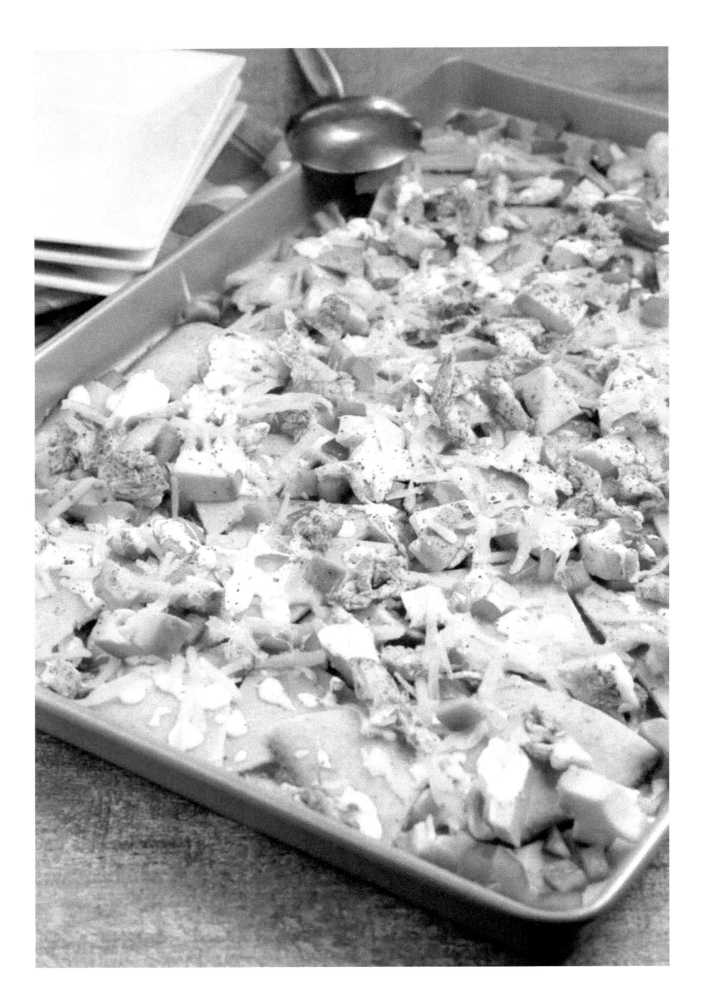

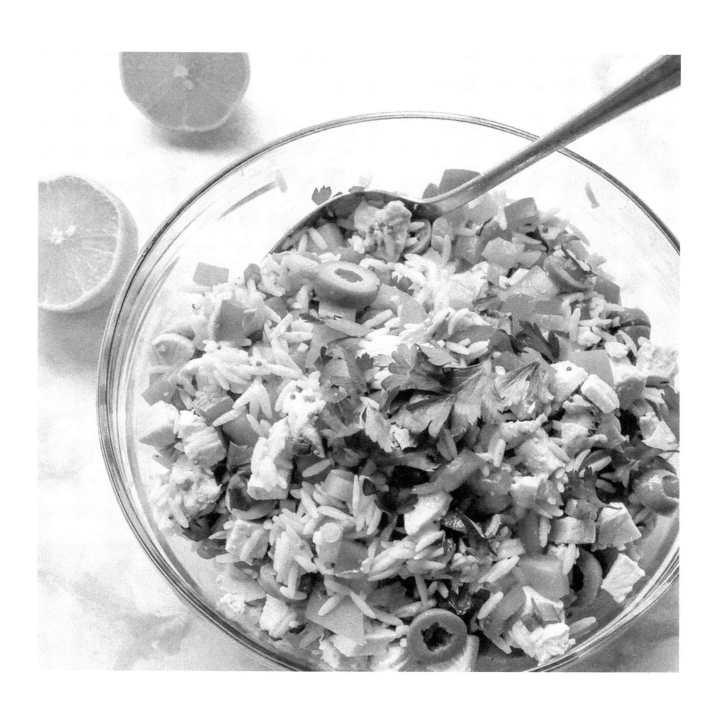

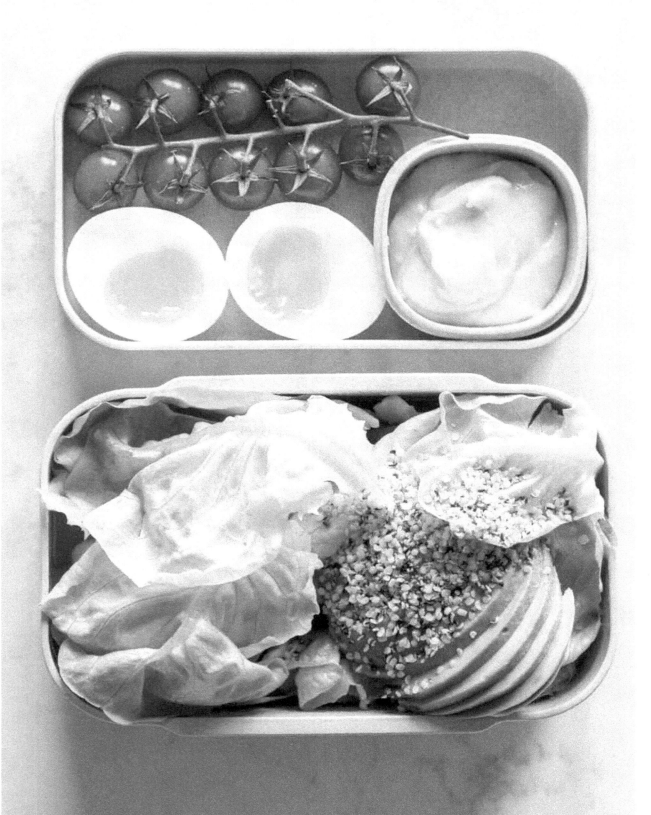